MW00513537

Mediterranean Diet Cookbook for Beginners

– Flavorful and Healthy Mediterranean Recipes for Novices –

[Pamela Hartley]

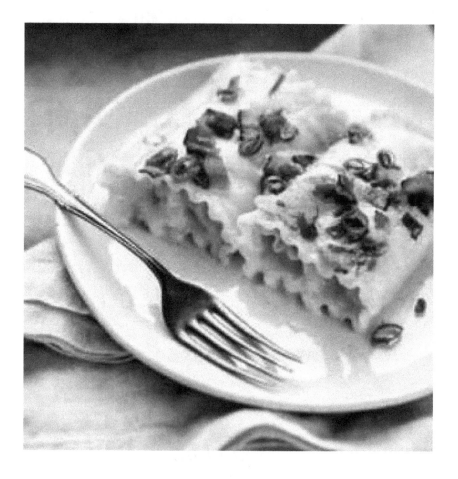

Table Of Content

CHAPTER 1: BREAKFAST **8**

    COCOA OATMEAL 8

    SPINACH OMELET 10

    RICOTTA TOAST 12

    AVOCADO MILK SHAKE 14

    FRUITY OATS... 15

    PEPERONI ROASTED IN OIL 17

    GOAT CHEESE FRITTATA CUPS 19

    YOGURT AND GRANOLA 21

    PEACH SMOOTHIE... 22

    CHIA SEEDS JAM 23

CHAPTER 2: LUNCH **25**

    TURKEY LASAGNA.. 26

    BAKED FISH ON LEMONS 28

    AVOCADO GAZPACHO 30

    GARLIC AIOLI... 32

    ARUGULA SALAD.. 34

    BULGARIAN MOUSSAKA.. 36

    RED ONION TILAPIA 39

    ORZO PRIMAVERA... 41

    RED WINE RISOTTO 43

    ZOODLES 45

    PANTRY PUTTANESCA 47

CHAPTER 3: DINNER **49**

    VEAL ROAST... 49

    LAMB SHANK 51

    ANCHOVY PASTA MANIA... 53

    POTATO SOUP 55

    EGYPTIAN KOSHARI 57

    BROWN BUTTER PERCH 59

    CREAMY CARROT SOUP 61

    SLAW... 63

    HADDOCK MARINARA.. 65

HALIBUT PAN 67

WRAPPED SCALLOPS 69

DUCK SAUCE... 71

LAMB RIBS.. 73

TOMATO AND FETA SALAD 75

CHAPTER 4: SNACK RECIPES **76**

CHOCOLATE OATMEAL COOKIES.. 76

BAKED APRICOT 78

ZUCCHINI CHIPS.. 79

BABA GANOUSH 81

SPICY ROASTED POTATOES 83

CHAPTER 5: DESSERTS..**85**

PEANUT CLUSTERS... 85

STRAWBERRIES WITH BALSAMIC VINEGAR 87

NUTMEG CAKE 88

COCONUT APPLES.. 91

CITRUS CHEESECAKE 93

STRAWBERRIES CREAM.. 96

SWEET RICE PUDDING 98

BROWNIE POPS 100

BLACK FOREST 103

PEAR JAM 105

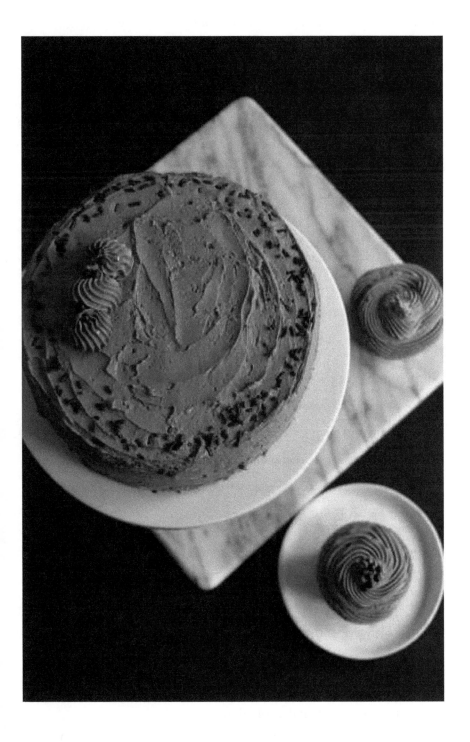

The following Book is reproduced below with the goal of providing information that is as accurate and reliable as possible. Regardless, purchasing this Book can be seen as consent to the fact that both the publisher and the author of this book are in no way experts on the topics discussed within and that any recommendations or suggestions that are made herein are for entertainment purposes only. Professionals should be consulted as needed prior to undertaking any of the action endorsed herein.

This declaration is deemed fair and valid by both the American Bar Association and the Committee of Publishers Association and is legally binding throughout the United States.

Furthermore, the transmission, duplication, or reproduction of any of the following work including specific information will be considered an illegal act irrespective of if it is done electronically or in print. This extends to creating a secondary or tertiary copy of the work or a recorded copy and is only allowed with the express written consent from the Publisher. All additional right reserved.

The information in the following pages is broadly considered a truthful and accurate account of facts and as such, any inattention, use, or misuse of the information in question by the reader will render any resulting actions solely under their purview. There are no scenarios in which the publisher or the original author of this work can be in any fashion deemed liable for any hardship or damages that may befall them after undertaking information described herein.

Additionally, the information in the following pages is intended only for informational purposes and should thus be thought of as universal. As befitting its nature, it is presented without assurance regarding its prolonged validity or interim quality. Trademarks that are mentioned are done without written consent and can in no way be considered an endorsement from the trademark holder.

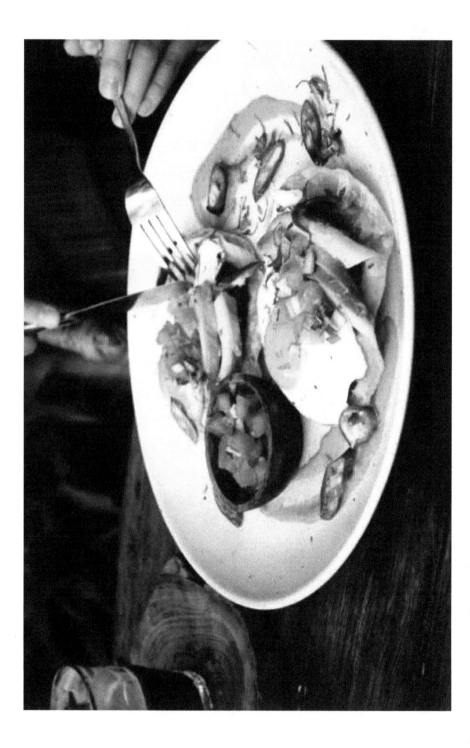

CHAPTER 1: BREAKFAST

Cocoa Oatmeal

Prep:

10 mins

Cook:

25 mins

Total:

35 mins

Servings:

4

Yield:

4 servings

Ingredients

1 ½ cups steel-cut oats
1 cup water
2 cups milk
3 tablespoons ground flax seed
1 ½ tablespoons cocoa powder
2 cups water
1 banana, mashed
¼ teaspoon nutmeg
⅓ cup walnut halves
1 teaspoon cinnamon

Directions

1

Stir 2 cups water, milk, and oats together in a large saucepan; bring to a boil. Reduce heat to medium-low and cook oats at a simmer until softened and beginning to thicken, about 15 minutes.

2

Stir 1 cup water, mashed banana, flax seed, cocoa powder, cinnamon, and nutmeg through the oats; continue cooking at a simmer until thick, about 8- 10 minutes. Fold walnuts into the oatmeal.

Nutrition
Per Serving:

413 calories; protein 14.8g; carbohydrates 57.5g; fat 15.3g; cholesterol 9.8mg; sodium 57.9mg.

Spinach Omelet

Prep:

6 mins

Cook:

9 mins

Total:

15 mins

Servings:

1

Yield:

1 serving

Ingredients

2 eggs
1 ½ tablespoons grated Parmesan cheese
¼ teaspoon onion powder
1 cup torn baby spinach leaves
salt and pepper to taste
⅛ teaspoon ground nutmeg

Directions

1

In a bowl, beat the eggs, and stir in the baby spinach and
Parmesan cheese. Season with onion powder, nutmeg, salt,
and pepper.

2

In a small skillet coated with cooking spray over medium heat,
cook the egg mixture about 3 minutes, until partially set. Flip

with a spatula, and continue cooking 2 to 4 minutes. Reduce heat to low, and continue cooking 2 to 4 minutes.

Nutrition
Per Serving:

186 calories; protein 16.4g; carbohydrates 2.8g; fat 12.3g; cholesterol 378.6mg; sodium 278.7mg.

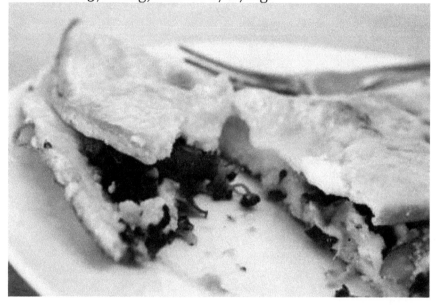

Ricotta Toast

Prep:

10 mins

Cook:

10 mins

Additional:

5 mins

Total:

25 mins

Servings:

2

Yield:

2 servings

Ingredients

1 teaspoon olive oil

1 large nectarine, pitted and cut into 8 wedges

2 thick slices crusty bread

2 tablespoons olive oil

¼ cup whole-milk ricotta cheese

1 tablespoon crushed sliced almonds

2 leaves fresh mint, minced

2 teaspoons honey, or to taste

Directions

1

Preheat an outdoor grill for medium-high heat and lightly oil grate.

2

Drizzle 1 teaspoon olive oil onto a small plate. Place nectarine wedges on the plate and cover all sides with oil. Brush both sides of bread with 2 tablespoons olive oil.

3

Place nectarines onto the hot grate and grill 1 to 3 minutes per side; remove to a plate. When nectarine wedges have cooled slightly, cut each wedge in 1/2 lengthwise so you now have 16 pieces.

4

Place bread slices onto the hot grate and cook until grill marks appear and bread is toasted, about 1 minute 30 seconds per side; remove to a plate.

5

Spread ricotta cheese onto each slice of toast. Arrange 8 nectarine slices onto each toast and top with almonds. Sprinkle with mint and drizzle with honey. Cut each toast in half and serve.

Nutrition Per Serving:

336 calories; protein 7.3g; carbohydrates 31.7g; fat 20.9g; cholesterol 8.8mg; sodium 199.8mg.

Avocado Milk Shake

Prep:

10 mins

Total:

10 mins

Servings:

2

Yield:

2 shakes

Ingredients

1 ripe avocado, peeled and chopped
4 pods cardamom pods
6 teaspoons white sugar, or to taste
2 cups cold milk

Directions

1

Pop cardamom pods open and crush or grind seeds into a powder.

2

Combine cardamom, milk, avocado, sugar, and salt in a food processor. Blend until smooth.

Nutrition
Per Serving:

332 calories; protein 10.1g; carbohydrates 32.6g; fat 19.5g; cholesterol 19.5mg; sodium 184.6mg.

Fruity Oats

Prep:

10 mins

Cook:

30 mins

Total:

40 mins

Servings:

12

Yield:

1 9-inch pan

Ingredients

1 ¼ cups all-purpose flour
½ cup butter
¾ cup fruit preserves
½ cup chocolate chips
⅓ cup white sugar
¼ cup honey
¾ cup quick-cooking oats
⅓ cup sliced almonds
2 tablespoons butter

Directions

1

Preheat the oven to 350 degrees F. Grease a 9-inch square pan.

2

Mix flour, 1/2 cup butter, and sugar together until combined. Spread over the bottom of the prepared pan.

3

Bake in the preheated oven until light golden brown, 16 to 20 minutes.

4

Mix preserves and chocolate chips in a bowl.

5

Combine honey and 2 tablespoons butter in a saucepan over medium heat; cook and stir until melted. Stir in oats and almonds.

6

Spread preserve mixture on top of the partially baked crust, then top with the oat mixture. Bake until lightly browned, about 20 minutes. Let cool before cutting into bars.

Nutrition
Per Serving:

299 calories; protein 3g; carbohydrates 43.3g; fat 13.5g; cholesterol 25.4mg; sodium 76.1mg.

Peperoni Roasted in Oil

Prep:

10 mins

Cook:

20 mins

Total:

30 mins

Servings:

6

Yield:

6 servings

Ingredients

1 red bell pepper
5 leaves fresh basil leaves, finely sliced
1 orange bell pepper
¾ cup extra-virgin olive oil
1 yellow bell pepper
1 clove garlic, minced
½ teaspoon salt
¼ teaspoon ground black pepper
½ teaspoon dried oregano

Directions

1

Preheat an outdoor grill for high heat and lightly oil the grate. Reduce grill heat to medium.

2

Grill whole peppers until charred on all sides, turning about every 5 minutes. Place charred peppers in a plastic food storage bag and tie shut. Allow peppers to cool in bag.

3

Combine olive oil, garlic, basil, oregano, salt, and pepper in a 1-pint glass jar (or larger, depending on size of peppers).

4

Remove cooled peppers from bag and scrape off charred skins. Cut peppers in half and remove seeds and stems. Slice peppers into long strips and place in oil mixture. Mix well, assuring peppers are covered in oil. Serve, storing leftover peppers in refrigerator for up to 5 days.

**Nutrition
Per Serving:**

270 calories; protein 0.7g; carbohydrates 4g; fat 28.2g; sodium 195.5mg.

Goat Cheese Frittata Cups

Prep:

15 mins

Cook:

10 mins

Total:

25 mins

Servings:

30

Yield:

30 cups

Ingredients

2 eggs, beaten

¼ cup finely grated Parmigiano-Reggiano cheese

salt and ground black pepper to taste

2 (1.9 ounce) packages frozen miniature phyllo cups (such as Athen's®)

5 ounces goat cheese

1 (10 ounce) box frozen chopped spinach, thawed and drained

Directions

1

Preheat the oven to 350 degrees F.

2

Combine goat cheese, eggs, and Parmigiano-Reggiano cheese in a medium bowl with a spoon or fork. Add spinach and season with salt and pepper.

3

Space phyllo cups evenly on an ungreased cookie sheet. Spoon 1 heaping teaspoonful of the cheese mixture into each cup, pressing a bit to fit it in; mixture will not expand during baking.

4

Bake in the preheated oven until filling is hot and phyllo cups are lightly browned, 10 to 12 minutes. Serve warm.

Nutrition
Per Serving:

47 calories; protein 2.4g; carbohydrates 2.8g; fat 2.8g; cholesterol 15.2mg; sodium 59.8mg.

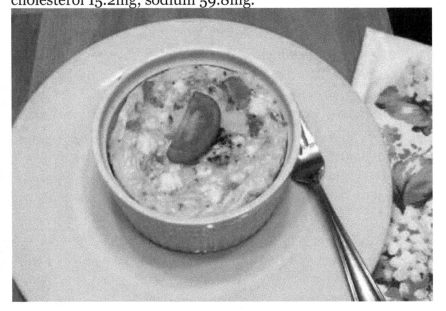

Yogurt and Granola

Prep:

5 mins

Total:

5 mins

Servings:

1

Yield:

1 serving

Ingredients

¼ cup granola
1 tablespoon light agave syrup
1 (6 ounce) container fat-free plain yogurt
1 pinch ground cinnamon, or to taste
1 tablespoon flaxseed meal

Directions

1

Stir yogurt, granola, agave syrup, flaxseed meal, and cinnamon together in a bowl.

Nutrition
Per Serving:

344 calories; protein 15.6g; carbohydrates 48.1g; fat 10.6g; cholesterol 3.4mg; sodium 140.7mg.

Peach Smoothie

Prep:

5 mins

Total:

5 mins

Servings:

1

Yield:

1 smoothie

Ingredients

1 large peach, sliced and frozen
½ cup soy milk
½ cup orange juice
1 banana, cut into pieces and frozen

Directions

1

Blend peach, banana, orange juice, soy milk, and flax seed in a blender until smooth.

Nutrition
Per Serving:

297 calories; protein 7.4g; carbohydrates 57.5g; fat 5.7g; sodium 71.7mg.

Chia Seeds Jam

Prep:

10 mins

Cook:

15 mins

Additional:

10 mins

Total:

35 mins

Servings:

10

Yield:

10 servings

Ingredients

½ cup water
2 cups frozen raspberries
¼ cup chia seeds
½ cup frozen blackberries
2 frozen strawberries, or more to taste
⅓ cup honey
½ cup frozen blueberries

Directions

1

Soak chia seeds in water until mixture has a jelly-like texture, about 6 minutes.

2

Heat raspberries, blackberries, blueberries, strawberries, and honey in a saucepan over medium heat until berries are soft, about 15 minutes. Lightly crush berries with a fork or masher.

3

Stir chia seed mixture into berry mixture. Remove from heat and let cool for at least 10 minutes.

Nutrition
Per Serving:

70 calories; protein 1g; carbohydrates 15.3g; fat 1g; sodium 1.9mg.

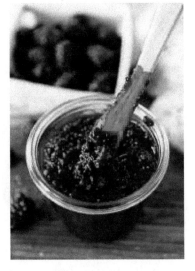

CHAPTER 2: LUNCH

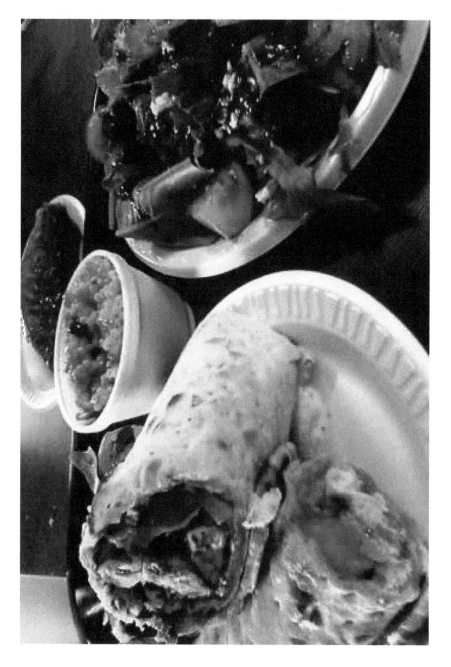

Turkey Lasagna

Servings:

4

Yield:

4 servings

Ingredients

1 onion, chopped
2 stalks celery, chopped
1 (16 ounce) package instant lasagna noodles
1 tablespoon vegetable oil
2 cups cooked and chopped turkey
½ teaspoon minced garlic
2 tablespoons butter
¼ cup all-purpose flour
salt to taste
ground black pepper to taste
1 cup cooked chopped broccoli
1 ½ cups milk
1 cup shredded mozzarella cheese

Directions

1

In a medium skillet saute the chopped onions, celery and garlic in oil until soft and tender. Add chopped turkey and broccoli. Set aside.

2

To make white sauce: In a small saucepan over low heat melt butter or margarine. Remove from heat and add flour, salt, and pepper; and blend well. Return to low heat, whisk in milk and cook until thick.

3

To assemble, in the bottom of a casserole dish place a thin layer of white sauce, then a layer of noodles. Next, place a layer of the turkey mixture, followed by sauce, and then 1/2 cup of the shredded mozzarella cheese. Repeat layering process with turkey mixture and sauce. Top with the remaining 1/2 cup of mozzarella cheese.

4

Bake in a preheated 350 degree oven for 45-55 minutes until bubbly and heated through. Let stand 12 to 15 minutes before serving.

Nutrition
Per Serving:

655 calories; protein 39.8g; carbohydrates 62.2g; fat 27.3g; cholesterol 107.1mg; sodium 341mg.

Baked Fish on Lemons

Prep:

10 mins

Cook:

15 mins

Total:

25 mins

Servings:

4

Yield:

4 servings

Ingredients

1 serving cooking spray

2 tablespoons dried parsley

2 pounds tilapia fillets, cut into serving-sized pieces

2 teaspoons lemon zest

¼ cup melted butter

½ teaspoon garlic powder

1 cup dry seasoned bread crumbs

Directions

1

Preheat the oven to 350 degrees F. Spray a baking dish with cooking spray.

2

Place tilapia pieces into the prepared baking dish. Combine bread crumbs, parsley, lemon zest, and garlic powder in a small bowl. Mix in melted butter and sprinkle mixture over fish fillets.

3

Bake in preheated oven until tilapia flakes easily with a fork, about 12-15 minutes.

Nutrition

Per Serving:

439 calories; protein 50.6g; carbohydrates 20.2g; fat 16.1g; cholesterol 113.8mg; sodium 383.7mg.

Avocado Gazpacho

Prep:

30 mins

Additional:

3 hrs

Total:

3 hrs 30 mins

Servings:

8

Yield:

8 servings

Ingredients

2 ½ cups tomato-vegetable juice cocktail (such as V8®)

3 large tomatoes, diced

½ cup chopped green bell pepper

3 large avocados - peeled, pitted, and cut into bite-sized pieces

1 cup diced cucumber

2 ½ cups vegetable broth

1 (8 ounce) can chopped tomatoes with juice

¼ cup extra-virgin olive oil

3 green onions, thinly sliced

1 lemon, juiced, or more to taste

2 tablespoons minced fresh cilantro

½ cup chopped red bell pepper

1 dash hot pepper sauce (such as Tabasco®), or to taste

2 tablespoons white wine vinegar

salt and ground black pepper to taste

Directions

1

Mix tomato-vegetable juice, vegetable broth, tomatoes, avocados, cucumber, canned tomatoes with juice, green bell pepper, red bell pepper, olive oil, green onions, lemon juice, cilantro, vinegar, hot pepper sauce, salt, and black pepper together in a large bowl. Cover and chill for at least 3 hours before serving to allow flavors to blend.

Nutrition

Per Serving:

287 calories; protein 4.5g; carbohydrates 21g; fat 23.1g; sodium 392.2mg.

Garlic Aioli

Prep:

10 mins

Cook:

1 hr

Additional:

1 hr 35 mins

Total:

2 hrs 45 mins

Servings:

4

Yield:

1 /2 cup

Ingredients

1 head garlic

kosher salt and ground black pepper to taste

1 pinch ground cayenne pepper

½ cup mayonnaise

1 teaspoon lemon juice

2 teaspoons olive oil

½ teaspoon Worcestershire sauce

Directions

1

Preheat oven to 350 degrees F.

2

Trim off the top of the head of garlic to expose cloves. Drizzle with olive oil. Sprinkle salt and black pepper on top. Wrap in aluminum foil.

3

Bake in the preheated oven until garlic feels soft when lightly pressed, about 1 hour. Unwrap and cool, 5 to 10 minutes. Refrigerate until chilled, 30 minutes to 1 hour.

4

Pull out individual garlic cloves with a sharp knife; place in a small bowl. Mash with a fork until creamy. Add mayonnaise, lemon juice, Worcestershire sauce, and cayenne; mix well until blended.

5

Refrigerate until flavors combine, at least 1 hour.

Nutrition

Per Serving:

240 calories; protein 1.1g; carbohydrates 5.8g; fat 24.3g; cholesterol 10.4mg; sodium 204.4mg.

Arugula Salad

Prep:

15 mins

Total:

15 mins

Servings:

4

Yield:

4 servings

Ingredients

4 cups young arugula leaves, rinsed and dried

1 large avocado - peeled, pitted and sliced

¼ cup grated Parmesan cheese

1 cup cherry tomatoes, halved

¼ cup pine nuts

1 tablespoon rice vinegar

salt to taste

2 tablespoons grapeseed oil or olive oil

freshly ground black pepper to taste

Directions

1

In a large plastic bowl with a lid, combine arugula, cherry tomatoes, pine nuts, oil, vinegar, and Parmesan cheese. Season with salt and pepper to taste. Cover, and shake to mix.

2

Divide salad onto plates, and top with slices of avocado.

Nutrition
Per Serving:

257 calories; protein 6.2g; carbohydrates 10g; fat 23.2g; cholesterol 4. 4mg; sodium 381.3mg.

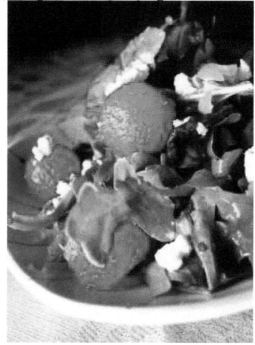

Bulgarian Moussaka

Prep:

30 mins

Cook:

1 hr 30 mins

Total:

2 hrs

Servings:

12

Yield:

12 servings

Ingredients

¾ pound ground beef (85% lean)

¾ pound ground pork

1 large carrot, finely chopped

½ yellow onion, finely chopped

½ cup olive oil, divided

2 stalks celery, finely chopped

1 (14.5 ounce) can diced tomatoes

1 red bell pepper, finely chopped

¼ bunch fresh parsley, stems and leaves chopped separately

2 tablespoons paprika

1 tablespoon salt

2 bay leaves

½ teaspoon cayenne pepper

1 teaspoon black pepper

6 russet potatoes, peeled and cut into 1/2-inch dice

Topping:

2 eggs

2 cups plain yogurt

1 teaspoon baking soda
¼ cup all-purpose flour

Directions

1

Heat a large skillet over medium heat. Add ground beef and
ground pork and cook until brown and crumbly, 5 to 10
minutes. Drain and discard fat. Add 1/4 cup olive oil, carrot,
onion, celery, parsley stems, and tomatoes. Mix to combine.
Stir in bell pepper and season with paprika, salt, pepper, bay
leaves, and cayenne pepper. Cook until vegetables start to
soften, about 10 minutes.

2

Meanwhile, preheat the oven to 400 degrees F.

3

Transfer meat mixture to a large baking pan.

4

Heat remaining 1/4 cup olive oil in a large skillet and cook
potatoes until lightly browned, about 10 minutes. Transfer to
the baking pan and mix well with the meat mixture.

5

Bake moussaka in the preheated oven for 45 minutes. Remove
baking dish from the oven and mix in chopped parsley leaves.

6

Stir eggs, yogurt, flour, and baking soda together in a bowl
until it turns into a spreadable mixture. Pour over the meat
mixture in the baking dish.

7
Return baking dish to the oven and cook until the top is golden brown, about 15 more minutes.

Nutrition
Per Serving:

335 calories; protein 16.4g; carbohydrates 27.7g; fat 17.8g; cholesterol 72.4mg; sodium 829.4mg.

Red Onion Tilapia

Prep:

10 mins

Cook:

15 mins

Additional:

2 mins

Total:

27 mins

Servings:

1

Yield:

1 tilapia fillet

Ingredients

¼ large lemon
salt and ground black pepper to taste
1 tablespoon grated fresh Parmesan cheese
1 tablespoon extra-virgin olive oil
1 (6 ounce) tilapia fillet, patted dry
1 teaspoon butter, divided
1 teaspoon minced garlic
¼ large red onion, coarsely chopped

Directions

1

Squeeze lemon juice over tilapia; season lightly with salt and
black pepper.

2

Heat olive oil in a nonstick skillet over medium heat. Melt 1/2 teaspoon butter in hot oil. Add chopped onion and minced garlic; cook and stir until onion begins to look translucent, about 5 minutes.

3

Reduce heat to medium-low. Push onion mixture to sides of the skillet. Melt remaining 1/2 teaspoon of butter in the skillet. Place tilapia in the center of the skillet and cover with onion mixture. Cover skillet and cook tilapia until it starts to turn golden, about 5 minutes. Push onion mixture to the sides again and flip tilapia. Cover and cook until second side is golden and flakes easily with a fork, about 5 minutes more.

4

Remove skillet from heat. Top tilapia with grated Parmesan cheese, cover, and let stand until cheese is melted, about 3 minutes.

Nutrition

Per Serving:

371 calories; protein 37.3g; carbohydrates 7.6g; fat 21.4g; cholesterol 76.7mg; sodium 337.8mg.

Orzo Primavera

Prep:

15 mins

Cook:

30 mins

Total:

45 mins

Servings:

6

Yield:

6 servings

Ingredients

4 teaspoons kosher salt, divided
1 tablespoon olive oil
1 red bell pepper, chopped
½ cup grated Parmesan cheese
1 ⅓ cups uncooked orzo pasta
1 carrot, cut into thin slices
1 tablespoon minced garlic
1 medium zucchini, cut into bite-sized pieces
1 medium onion, chopped
½ cup chicken broth
½ cup tomato sauce
¼ teaspoon ground black pepper
2 tablespoons half-and-half
1 medium yellow squash, cut into bite-sized pieces

Directions

1

Bring a large pot of water to a rolling boil; add 2 teaspoons salt. Cook orzo in the boiling water, stirring occasionally until tender yet firm to the bite, 6 to 10 minutes. Drain.

2

Heat oil in a skillet over low heat. Add bell pepper and saute for 10 minutes. Increase heat to medium and add carrot, onion, and garlic. Saute until carrot begins to soften, about 3 minutes. Add zucchini and summer squash; cook for 1 minute more. Increase heat to high and add broth, tomato sauce, remaining salt, and pepper. Cook until sauce comes to a simmer, about 5 minutes. Reduce heat to low.

3

Add orzo to the sauce and mix well. Remove from heat. Stir in half-and-half, followed by Parmesan cheese. Serve hot or at room temperature.

Nutrition

Per Serving: 253 calories; protein 10.4g; carbohydrates 41.3g; fat 5.7g; cholesterol 8.2mg; sodium 1602.7mg.

Red Wine Risotto

Prep:

10 mins

Cook:

30 mins

Total:

40 mins

Servings:

4

Yield:

4 servings

Ingredients

2 tablespoons olive oil

1 ½ ounces prosciutto

1 large shallot, minced

2 chanterelle mushrooms, sliced

1 cup arborio rice

1 cup red wine

1 clove garlic, chopped

3 cups beef stock, or more as needed, divided

½ cup arugula

1 tablespoon chopped fresh thyme

ground black pepper to taste

⅓ cup freshly grated Parmesan cheese

Directions

1

Heat olive oil in a Dutch oven or heavy pot over medium heat; cook prosciutto until edges begin to curl and fat is rendered, 2 to 3 minutes. Add shallot and cook until fragrant, about 2 minutes. Add garlic and cook until fragrant, about 1 minute. Add mushrooms and cook for 30 seconds.

2

Cook and stir rice into prosciutto mixture, stirring continually, until rice is translucent around edges, 1 to 2 minutes. Pour red wine into rice mixture; cook, stirring every 30 seconds, until wine is absorbed, about 5 minutes. Stir 1 cup broth into rice mixture, cooking and stirring until broth is almost completely absorbed, 4-5 minutes. Continue adding 1 cup broth at a time, stirring constantly, until rice is tender, 15 to 20 minutes.

3

Mix arugula, Parmesan cheese, thyme, and black pepper into rice mixture; cook and stir until cheese is melted, 2 to 4 minutes.

Nutrition
Per Serving:

408 calories; protein 11.8g; carbohydrates 48.7g; fat 12.9g; cholesterol 15.2mg; sodium 380.5mg.

Zoodles

Prep:
10 mins

Cook:
10 mins

Total:
20 mins

Servings:
2

Yield:
2 servings

Ingredients

1 tablespoon olive oil
½ cup drained and rinsed canned garbanzo beans (chickpeas)
3 tablespoons pesto, or to taste
2 tablespoons shredded white Cheddar cheese
4 small zucchini, cut into noodle-shape strands
salt and ground black pepper to taste

Directions

1

Heat olive oil in a skillet over medium heat; cook and stir zucchini until tender and liquid has evaporated, 6 to 10 minutes.

2

Stir garbanzo beans and pesto into zucchini; lower heat to medium-low. Cook and stir until garbanzo beans are warm and zucchini is evenly coated, about 5 minutes; season with salt and pepper.

3
Transfer zucchini mixture to serving bowls and top with white Cheddar cheese.

Nutrition
Per Serving:

319 calories; protein 12.1g; carbohydrates 23.1g; fat 21.3g; cholesterol 16.2mg; sodium 510.8mg.

Pantry Puttanesca

Prep:

5 mins

Cook:

16 mins

Total:

21 mins

Servings:

4

Yield:

4 servings

Ingredients

⅓ cup olive oil

3 cloves garlic, minced

½ cup chopped pitted kalamata olives

1 teaspoon dried oregano

3 anchovy fillets, chopped

2 (15 ounce) cans diced tomatoes, drained.

1 (8 ounce) package spaghetti

¼ cup capers, chopped

¼ teaspoon crushed red pepper flakes

Directions

1

Fill a large pot with water. Bring to a rolling boil over high heat.

2

As the water heats, pour the olive oil into a cold skillet and stir in the garlic. Turn heat to medium-low and cook and stir until the garlic is fragrant and begins to turn a golden color, 1 to 2 minutes. Stir in the red pepper flakes, oregano, and anchovies. Cook until anchovies begin to break down, about 2 minutes.

3

Pour tomatoes into skillet, turn heat to medium-high, and bring sauce to a simmer. Use the back of a spoon to break down tomatoes as they cook. Simmer until sauce is reduced and combined, about 10-12 minutes.

4

Meanwhile, cook the pasta in the boiling water. Drain when still very firm to the bite, about 10 minutes. Reserve 1/2 cup pasta water.

5

Stir the olives and capers into the sauce; add pasta and toss to combine.

6

Toss pasta in sauce until pasta is cooked through and well coated with sauce, about 1 minute. If sauce becomes too thick, stir in some of the reserved pasta water to thin.

Nutrition

Per Serving:

463 calories; protein 10.5g; carbohydrates 53.3g; fat 24g; cholesterol 2.5mg; sodium 944.5mg.

CHAPTER 3: DINNER

Veal Roast

Prep:

1 hr

Cook:

1 hr 30 mins

Total:

2 hrs 30 mins

Servings:

8

Yield:

8 servings

Ingredients

4 pounds veal shoulder roast

4 carrots, halved

½ pound small white onions

¼ teaspoon dried thyme

½ pound mushrooms

1 pound small potatoes

1 (10 ounce) package frozen green peas

2 egg yolks

2 tablespoons all-purpose flour

Directions

1

In an 8 quart Dutch oven over medium-high heat, brown roast on all sides. Add thyme and 2 cups of water. Heat to boiling, then reduce heat to low, cover, and simmer 30 minutes.

2

To the pot, add carrots, potatoes and onions. Cover, and simmer 30 minutes. Toss in mushrooms. Cover, and simmer 15 minutes, or until vegetables and veal are tender. Remove roast and vegetables, and keep warm.

3

In a cup, stir flour and 2 tablespoons water until blended with no lumps. Gradually stir into liquid in Dutch oven. Cook, stirring constantly, until gravy is slightly thickened. Stir in peas, and heat through.

4

In a small bowl, beat egg yolks. Stir in a small amount of hot gravy. Slowly pour egg yolk mixture back into gravy, whisking until thickened. IMPORTANT: DO NOT BOIL!
To serve, pour some gravy over the veal and vegetables. Serve remaining gravy in a gravy boat.

Nutrition

Per Serving: 414 calories; protein 48.9g; carbohydrates 23g; fat 13.3g; cholesterol 255.3mg; sodium 284.3mg.

Lamb Shank

Prep:

15 mins

Cook:

1 hr

Additional:

1 hr

Total:

2 hrs 15 mins

Servings:

6

Yield:

6 servings

Ingredients

1 (4 pound) lamb shank
Marinade:
¼ teaspoon ground thyme
¼ teaspoon dried basil
3 tablespoons olive oil
1 teaspoon dried rosemary
¼ teaspoon dried parsley
2 tablespoons ground black pepper
1 pinch salt to taste
½ teaspoon dried mint
Basting Sauce:
¼ cup lemon juice
3 tablespoons honey

Directions

1

Cut slits into lamb shank in a criss-cross pattern about 1 inch apart and 1/2 inch deep; place into a shallow dish.

2

Whisk olive oil, rosemary, thyme, basil, parsley, mint, black pepper, salt, and cayenne pepper together in a bowl; brush evenly over the lamb shank. Refrigerate lamb at least 1 hour.

3

Preheat grill for medium heat and lightly oil the grate.

4

Stir lemon juice and honey together in a small bowl until smooth.

5

Cook lamb shank on preheated grill, basting every 15 minutes with the lemon juice mixture, until browned on the outside and red in the center, about 30 minutes per side. An instant-read thermometer inserted into the center should read 125 degrees F.

Nutrition

Per Serving: 342 calories; protein 36.3g; carbohydrates 11.2g; fat 16.5g; cholesterol 109.8mg; sodium 93.3mg.

Anchovy Pasta Mania

Prep:

10 mins

Cook:

25 mins

Total:

35 mins

Servings:

2

Yield:

2 servings

Ingredients

1 head broccoli, cut into florets
1 pinch ground black pepper to taste
3 tablespoons olive oil, divided
2 pinches salt to taste
6 anchovy fillets in olive oil, drained
3 cloves garlic, thinly sliced
½ (16 ounce) package linguine pasta
½ teaspoon red pepper flakes, or more to taste

Directions

1

Set an oven rack about 8 inches from the heat source and preheat the oven's broiler. Toss broccoli in a bowl with 1 tablespoon olive oil and salt; spread on a large baking sheet.

2

Broil in the preheated oven until broccoli is tender and beginning to brown, 5 to 10 minutes.

3

Bring a large pot of lightly salted water to a boil. Cook linguine at a boil until tender yet firm to the bite, approximately 11 minutes.

4

Heat 1 tablespoon olive oil in a large skillet over low heat. Add anchovies, garlic, and red pepper flakes; cook and stir until anchovies dissolve into the oil, 3 to 5 minutes. Season with pepper. Mix in roasted broccoli.

5

Drain pasta and return to the pot. Add broccoli-anchovy mixture and mix well. Drizzle remaining olive oil on top.

Nutrition
Per Serving: 667 calories; protein 23g; carbohydrates 93.7g; fat 24.7g; cholesterol 10.2mg; sodium 652.1mg.

Potato Soup

Servings:
9
Yield:
8 to 10 servings

Ingredients

8 unpeeled potatoes, cubed
1 onion, chopped
2 stalks celery, diced
6 cubes chicken bouillon
1 pound bacon - cooked and crumbled
1 (10.75 ounce) can condensed cream of mushroom soup
1 pint half-and-half cream
2 cups shredded Cheddar cheese

Directions
1

In a large stock pot combine potatoes, onions, celery, bouillon cubes and enough water to cover all **Ingredients**. Bring to a boil and simmer on medium heat until potatoes are with in 15 minutes of being finished.

2

Add half and half, bacon, cream of mushroom soup and stir until creamy. Add cheese and stir until completely melted. Simmer on low until potatoes are done.

Nutrition

Per Serving: 642 calories; protein 31.8g; carbohydrates 41.2g; fat 38.9g; cholesterol 105.3mg; sodium 2352.2mg.

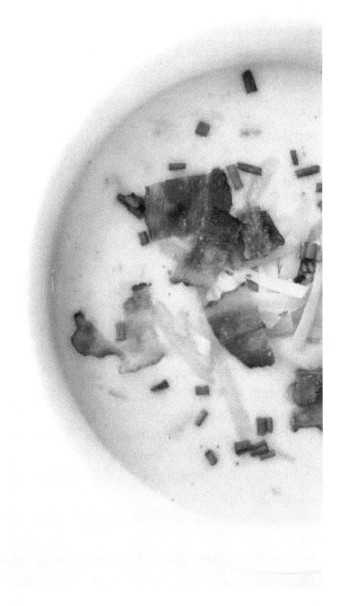

Egyptian Koshari

Prep:

15 mins

Cook:

45 mins

Total:

1 hr

Servings:

4

Yield:

4 servings

Ingredients

¾ cup brown lentils
¾ cup uncooked long grain rice
4 cups water
1 cup elbow macaroni
2 large onions, chopped
4 cloves garlic, minced
1 (15.5 ounce) can diced tomatoes
¼ teaspoon red pepper flakes
2 tablespoons vegetable oil
salt and pepper to taste

Directions

1

Combine the lentils and water in a large saucepan. Bring to a boil, then simmer over medium heat for 25 minutes. Add the rice to the lentils, and continue to simmer for an additional 20 minutes, or until rice is tender.

2

Fill a separate saucepan with lightly salted water and bring to a boil. Add the macaroni and cook until tender, about 8 minutes. Drain.

3

Meanwhile, heat the vegetable oil in a large skillet over medium heat. Add onion and garlic; cook and stir until onion is lightly browned. Pour in the tomatoes and season with red pepper flakes, salt and pepper. Simmer over medium heat for 10 to 20 minutes.

4

In a large serving dish, stir together the lentils, rice and macaroni. Mix in the tomato sauce until evenly coated.

Nutrition
Per Serving: 469 calories; protein 17.1g; carbohydrates 80.7g; fat 7.9g; sodium 186.5mg.

Brown Butter Perch

Prep:

10 mins

Cook:

10 mins

Total:

20 mins

Servings:

4

Yield:

4 servings

Ingredients

1 cup flour
1 lemon, cut in half
1 teaspoon salt
½ teaspoon cayenne pepper
8 ounces fresh perch fillets
½ teaspoon finely ground black pepper
2 tablespoons butter

Directions

1

Whisk flour, salt, black pepper, and cayenne pepper in a bowl. Gently press perch fillets into flour mixture to coat, shaking off any excess flour.

2

Heat butter in a skillet over medium heat until butter is foaming and nut-brown in color. Working in batches, place filets in skillet and cook until light golden, about 2 minutes per side. Transfer cooked fillets to a plate, squeeze lemon juice over the top, and serve.

Nutrition

Per Serving: 271 calories; protein 12.6g; carbohydrates 30.9g; fat 11.5g; cholesterol 43.2mg; sodium 702.8mg.

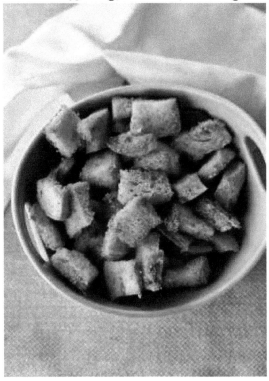

Creamy Carrot Soup

Prep:

10 mins

Cook:

35 mins

Total:

45 mins

Servings:

3

Yield:

3 cups

Ingredients

1 cup diced carrots
¼ cup chopped onion
¼ cup cubed potatoes
2 cups vegetable broth
½ teaspoon grated fresh ginger root
1 tablespoon butter
¼ cup heavy cream
salt and pepper to taste
2 ½ tablespoons chopped fresh dill

Directions

1

Melt butter in a small saucepan. Sweat the carrots, onion and ginger with the butter. Add potatoes and broth, then bring to a boil. Reduce heat, and simmer until potatoes are tender. Strain liquid into a separate container. Put vegetables into a blender along with the dill, and pour in just enough of the liquid to cover the vegetables. Puree in stages if necessary. Discard excess broth. Return vegetable puree to pan.

2

Stir heavy cream into the pan with the vegetables. Season with salt and pepper. Heat, but do not boil, and serve immediately.

Nutrition

Per Serving: 161 calories; protein 2.1g; carbohydrates 11.7g; fat 12.2g; cholesterol 39.2mg; sodium 373.1mg.

Slaw

Prep:

15 mins

Cook:

5 mins

Total:

20 mins

Servings:

8

Yield:

8 servings

Ingredients

¼ cup chopped pecans
1 tablespoon sugar
1 (8.5 ounce) package coleslaw mix
¼ cup crumbled feta cheese
½ cup mayonnaise
½ cup Ranch dressing
½ cup matchstick-style shredded carrots
1 ½ cups red grapes

Directions

1

In a medium ungreased skillet, over medium heat, toast the pecans by stirring frequently until golden brown. Set aside to cool.

2

In a large bowl, combine coleslaw mix, carrots, grapes, pecans, and feta cheese.

3
In a small bowl, stir together the mayonnaise, and Ranch
dressing. Pour in sugar, and mix until dissolved. Toss coleslaw
mixture with dressing until evenly coated. Serve immediately.

Nutrition
Per Serving: 265 calories; protein 2g; carbohydrates 13.2g; fat
23.4g; cholesterol 15.9mg; sodium 286.8mg.

Haddock Marinara

Prep:

15 mins

Cook:

30 mins

Total:

45 mins

Servings:

4

Yield:

4 servings

Ingredients

2 tablespoons extra virgin olive oil

¾ cup shredded mozzarella cheese

½ white onion, finely chopped

3 cloves garlic, minced

1 pound haddock fillets

1 (14 ounce) can stewed tomatoes, drained

1 (16 ounce) jar pasta sauce

Directions

1

Preheat oven to 350 degrees F. Coat the bottom of a baking
dish with the olive oil.

2

Sprinkle 1/2 the onion and garlic evenly in the baking dish,
and cover with 1/2 the pasta sauce. Place the haddock fillets in
the dish, top with tomatoes and remaining onion and garlic.
Cover with remaining pasta sauce.

3
Bake 20 minutes in the preheated oven. Top with mozzarella cheese, and continue baking 10 minutes, until cheese is melted and fish is easily flaked with a fork.

Nutrition
Per Serving: 345 calories; protein 29.8g; carbohydrates 24.1g; fat 14.2g; cholesterol 80.5mg; sodium 885mg.

Halibut Pan

Prep:

15 mins

Cook:

10 mins

Total:

25 mins

Servings:

4

Yield:

4 servings

Ingredients

1 egg

1 cup all-purpose flour

2 tablespoons olive oil

1 teaspoon seafood seasoning (such as Old Bay®)

ground black pepper

1 pound skinless, boneless halibut fillets

1 teaspoon salt

2 tablespoons dried herbes de Provence

Directions

1

Whisk egg in a small bowl.

2

Combine flour, herbes de Provence, seafood seasoning, salt, and black pepper in a separate small bowl.

3

Cut halibut into 4 equal pieces.

4

Heat olive oil in a large frying pan over medium-low heat.

5

Dip each piece of halibut in whisked egg.

6

Dredge all sides of each piece in flour mixture to evenly coat; tap off excess flour.

7

Place coated pieces immediately in the hot olive oil.

8

Cook the halibut until lightly browned, about 5 minutes; turn and cook until fish is opaque and flakes easily with a fork, another 2 minutes.

Nutrition

Per Serving: 323 calories; protein 29.1g; carbohydrates 25.5g; fat 10.5g; cholesterol 83.1mg; sodium 787mg.

Wrapped Scallops

Prep:

15 mins

Cook:

10 mins

Total:

25 mins

Servings:

5

Yield:

10 appetizers

Ingredients

10 slices bacon
10 sea scallops
1 tablespoon olive oil
1 lemon, cut into wedges
1 teaspoon Cajun seasoning

Directions

1

Arrange bacon in a large skillet and cook over medium-high heat, turning occasionally, until lightly browned but still pliable, about 5 minutes. Drain the bacon slices on paper towels.

2

Wrap each slice of bacon around one sea scallop and secure with a toothpick. Season with Cajun seasoning.

3
Heat olive oil in a clean skillet over medium-high heat; sear scallops until golden and bacon is crisp, 3 to 4 minutes on each side. Squeeze lemon over scallops. Serve immediately.

Nutrition

Per Serving: 198 calories; protein 21.1g; carbohydrates 3.1g; fat 10.9g; cholesterol 54.4mg; sodium 683mg

Duck Sauce

Prep:

20 mins

Cook:

40 mins

Additional:

30 mins

Total:

1 hr 30 mins

Servings:

8

Yield:

8 Cups

Ingredients

5 cups coarsely chopped mixed fruit (apples, plums, and pears)
½ teaspoon dry mustard
1 cup water
1 teaspoon soy sauce
1 tablespoon apricot preserves
½ cup packed light brown sugar
½ teaspoon garlic powder
¾ cup apple juice

Directions

1

Place fruit in a stock pot over medium high heat. Add water, apple juice, soy sauce, apricot preserves, brown sugar, garlic powder, and dry mustard. Bring to a simmer, stirring frequently to dissolve brown sugar. Reduce heat, and continue simmering for 40 minutes, or until fruit is completely soft. Remove from heat and allow to cool.

2

Blend sauce in a food processor or blender until completely smooth, adjusting consistency with additional water, if desired. Cover, and refrigerate until ready to use.

Nutrition

Per Serving: 224 calories; protein 2.4g; carbohydrates 55.9g; fat 0.4g; sodium 47.6mg.

Lamb Ribs

Prep:

10 mins

Cook:

1 hr 10 mins

Additional:

1 hr

Total:

2 hrs 20 mins

Servings:

6

Yield:

6 servings

Ingredients

3 ½ pounds lamb ribs
1 teaspoon ground black pepper
2 onions, chopped
1 cup dry white wine
¼ cup soy sauce
¼ cup fresh lemon juice
1 tablespoon honey
1 tablespoon olive oil
2 teaspoons minced garlic
1 teaspoon ground cinnamon
1 teaspoon salt

Directions

1

Place lamb in a 9x13-inch baking dish.

2

Combine onions, white wine, soy sauce, lemon juice, honey, olive oil, garlic, cinnamon, salt, and pepper in a small bowl. Mix well and pour mixture all over lamb. Cover with plastic wrap and marinate in the refrigerator for 1 hour.

3

Preheat oven to 400 degrees F.

4

Roast lamb in the preheated oven until browned and tender, about 1 hour 10 minutes.

Nutrition

Per Serving: 508 calories; protein 25.8g; carbohydrates 10.2g; fat 36.8g; cholesterol 112.2mg; sodium 1077.1mg.

Tomato and Feta Salad

Prep:
10 mins
Total:
10 mins
Servings:
4
Yield:
4 servings

Ingredients

4 teaspoons white wine vinegar
2 tablespoons chopped fresh basil
4 teaspoons olive oil
1 pint cherry tomatoes, halved
2 tablespoons finely chopped shallot
¼ cup crumbled feta cheese
¼ teaspoon coarse salt

Directions
1
Whisk vinegar, olive oil, and salt in a salad bowl. Stir in cherry tomatoes, shallot, feta cheese, and basil.

Nutrition
Per Serving: 103 calories; protein 3g; carbohydrates 5g; fat 8.4g; cholesterol 14mg; sodium 329.1mg.

CHAPTER 4: SNACK RECIPES

Chocolate Oatmeal Cookies

Servings:

24

Yield:

4 dozen

Ingredients

½ cup milk

3 cups quick cooking oats

2 cups white sugar

½ cup peanut butter

5 tablespoons cocoa powder

½ cup butter

Directions

1

Cook butter or margarine, milk and sugar in kettle and boil for 1 and 1/2 minutes.

2

Add peanut butter, oatmeal, cocoa powder and any one of the optional **Ingredients**.

3

Drop on waxed paper and allow to cool before serving.

Nutrition

Per Serving: 207 calories; protein 3.6g; carbohydrates 29.3g; fat 9.5g; cholesterol 10.6mg; sodium 59.6mg.

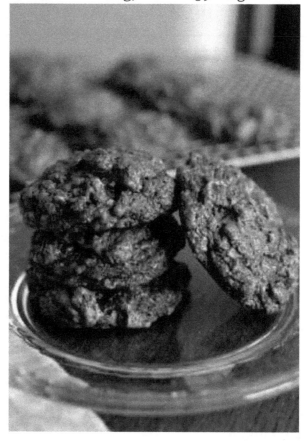

Baked Apricot

Servings:

6

Yield:

6 servings

Ingredients

3 (15 ounce) cans apricot halves, drained
50 buttery round crackers, crumbled
¾ cup packed brown sugar
½ cup butter, melted

Directions

1
Preheat oven to 325 degrees F.

2
In an 8x12 inch baking pan, layer half of apricots, brown sugar, cracker crumbs, and butter. Repeat.

3
Bake for 50 to 60 minutes.

Nutrition

Per Serving: 588 calories; protein 3.4g; carbohydrates 100g; fat 21.7g; cholesterol 61.5mg; sodium 341.9mg.

Zucchini Chips

Prep:

10 mins

Cook:

2 hrs

Total:

2 hrs 10 mins

Servings:

2

Yield:

2 servings

Ingredients

2 large large zucchini, thinly sliced
1 tablespoon olive oil, or to taste
sea salt to taste

Directions

1

Preheat oven to 250 degrees F.

2

Arrange sliced zucchini on a baking sheet. Drizzle lightly with olive oil and sprinkle lightly with sea salt.

3

Bake in the preheated oven until completely dried and chip-like, about 1 hour per side. Allow to cool before serving.

Nutrition

Per Serving: 111 calories; protein 3.9g; carbohydrates 10.8g; fat 7.3g; sodium 192.4mg.

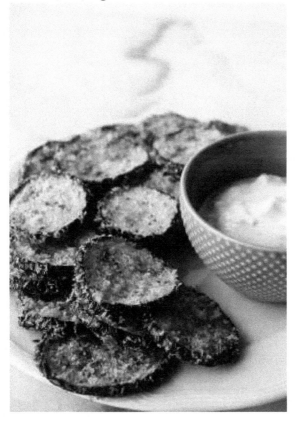

Baba Ganoush

Prep:

15 mins

Cook:

20 mins

Additional:

30 mins

Total:

1 hr 5 mins

Servings:

4

Yield:

4 servings

Ingredients

1 pound eggplant
2 tablespoons lemon juice
1 pinch paprika
2 tablespoons tahini
2 cloves garlic
⅛ teaspoon red chile powder
1 tablespoon extra-virgin olive oil
½ tablespoon plain yogurt
⅛ teaspoon ground cumin
salt to taste

Directions

1

Preheat the oven to 450 degrees F. Lightly oil a baking sheet.

2

Halve eggplants and brush cut sides with olive oil. Place face-down onto the prepared baking sheet.

3

Roast in the preheated oven until softened, 20 to 25 minutes. Remove from oven and let cool, about 30 minutes.

4

Scoop flesh out of skins and place in a mesh strainer. Discard skins. Press down on flesh to remove liquid or drippings. Transfer eggplant flesh to a food processor. Add lemon juice, tahini, garlic, cumin, and chile powder. Drizzle olive oil on top of everything. Blend well, 50 seconds to 1 minute.

5

Mix in plain yogurt and season with salt. Serve with a sprinkle of paprika over top for garnish.

Nutrition

Per Serving: 109 calories; protein 2.7g; carbohydrates 9.5g; fat 7.7g; cholesterol 0.1mg; sodium 51.5mg.

Spicy Roasted Potatoes

Prep:

15 mins

Cook:

40 mins

Total:

55 mins

Servings:

4

Yield:

4 servings

Ingredients

5 medium red potatoes, diced with peel
1 tablespoon garlic powder
1 tablespoon kosher salt
2 teaspoons chili powder
¼ cup extra virgin olive oil
1 medium onion, chopped

Directions

1

Preheat the oven to 450 degrees F.

2

Arrange the potatoes and onions in a greased 9x13 inch baking dish so that they are evenly distributed. Season with garlic powder, salt and chili powder. Drizzle with olive oil. Stir to coat potatoes and onions with oil and spices.

3

Bake for 35 to 40 minutes in the preheated oven, until potatoes are fork tender and slightly crispy. Stir every 10 minutes. When done, sprinkle with cheese. Wait about 5 minutes for the cheese to melt before serving.

Nutrition

Per Serving: 473 calories; protein 14.4g; carbohydrates 47.6g; fat 26.1g; cholesterol 36.2mg; sodium 1685.1mg.

CHAPTER 5: DESSERTS

Peanut Clusters

Servings:

12

Yield:

2 dozen

Ingredients

1 cup white sugar
¼ cup butter
¼ cup crunchy peanut butter
½ teaspoon vanilla extract
⅓ cup evaporated milk
2 cups quick cooking oats
3 (1 ounce) squares semisweet chocolate
½ cup peanuts

Directions

1

Line cookie sheet with waxed paper.

2

Mix sugar, milk and butter or margarine over low heat and bring to a boil. Remove from heat and add peanut butter and vanilla until blended. Stir in remaining **Ingredients**.

3
Drop by tablespoons onto cookie sheet. If mixture becomes too stiff, stir in 1 to 2 drops milk. Refrigerate about 30 minutes or until firm.

Nutrition
Per Serving: 262 calories; protein 5.5g; carbohydrates 33g; fat 13.2g; cholesterol 12.2mg; sodium 62mg.

Strawberries with Balsamic Vinegar

Prep:

10 mins

Additional:

1 hr

Total:

1 hr 10 mins

Servings:

6

Yield:

6 servings

Ingredients

16 ounces fresh strawberries, hulled and large berries cut in half

¼ cup white sugar

2 tablespoons balsamic vinegar

¼ teaspoon freshly ground black pepper, or to taste

Directions

1

Place strawberries in a bowl. Drizzle vinegar over strawberries, and sprinkle with sugar. Stir gently to combine. Cover, and let sit at room temperature for at least 1 hour but not more than 4 hours. Just before serving, grind pepper over berries.

Nutrition

Per Serving: 60 calories; protein 0.5g; carbohydrates 14.9g; fat 0.2g; sodium 2.1mg.

Nutmeg Cake

Prep:

35 mins

Cook:

25 mins

Additional:

2 hrs

Total:

3 hrs

Servings:

12

Yield:

2 9-inch layers

Ingredients

½ cup butter, softened
1 ½ cups white sugar
1 teaspoon baking soda
1 cup buttermilk
1 teaspoon vanilla extract
2 cups all-purpose flour
1 teaspoon baking powder
2 teaspoons ground nutmeg
¼ teaspoon salt
3 eggs, room temperature
Caramel Icing:
½ cup packed brown sugar
3 tablespoons cream
¼ cup butter

1 ½ cups confectioners' sugar

Directions

1

Preheat oven to 350 degrees F. Lightly grease two 9-inch round cake pans.

2

Beat the butter and white sugar with an electric mixer in a large bowl until light and fluffy. The mixture should be noticeably lighter in color. Add the room-temperature eggs in three batches, blending them into the butter mixture fully. Stir in the vanilla.

3

Sift together the flour, baking powder, baking soda, nutmeg, and salt.

4

Pour 1/3 of the flour mixture into the bowl; mix just until incorporated. Stir in 1/2 the buttermilk, mixing gently. Continue adding the flour alternately with the buttermilk, mixing until combined. Spread the batter into the prepared pans.

5

Bake in the preheated oven until a toothpick inserted in the center of the cakes comes out clean, about 25 to 30 minutes. Let the cakes cool in the pans for 10 minutes, then invert them on a wire rack to cool completely before icing.

6

To make the Caramel Icing: In a medium saucepan, heat the brown sugar, cream or milk, and 1/4 cup butter until it boils.

Boil for 2 minutes, then remove from heat. Let cool. Stir in confectioner's sugar and beat until smooth. Add more cream or milk or confectioner's sugar as needed to achieve desired spreading consistency. Makes about 1 1/3 cups.

Nutrition
Per Serving: 410 calories; protein 4.6g; carbohydrates 66.4g; fat 14.7g; cholesterol 82.9mg; sodium 319.3mg.

Coconut Apples

Prep:

25 mins

Cook:

30 mins

Total:

55 mins

Servings:

7

Yield:

1 large baking dish

Ingredients

½ cup caramel ice cream topping

¾ cup sweetened flaked coconut

1 tablespoon all-purpose flour

1 (10 ounce) can refrigerated flaky biscuit dough

4 Granny Smith apples - peeled, cored and sliced

2 tablespoons butter

3 tablespoons white sugar

Directions

1

Preheat oven to 375 degrees F .

2

Stir together apples, caramel topping, and flour in a large round baking dish. Pull apart each biscuit into two halves, and arrange over the apples. Drizzle with butter. Stir together the sugar and coconut; sprinkle over the buttered biscuits.

3

Bake in preheated oven until the biscuits have puffed, and are lightly browned, about 30 minutes.

Directions

1

Preheat oven to 375 degrees F .

2

Stir together apples, caramel topping, and flour in a large round baking dish. Pull apart each biscuit into two halves, and arrange over the apples. Drizzle with butter. Stir together the sugar and coconut; sprinkle over the buttered biscuits.

3

Bake in preheated oven until the biscuits have puffed, and are lightly browned, about 30 minutes.

Citrus Cheesecake

Prep:

30 mins

Cook:

1 hr 10 mins

Additional:

20 mins

Total:

2 hrs

Servings:

12

Yield:

1 - 9 inch springform pan

Ingredients

1 egg yolk
1 tablespoon fresh lemon juice
1 egg white
3 (8 ounce) packages cream cheese
1 teaspoon grated lemon zest
¼ teaspoon vanilla extract
⅓ cup white sugar
½ cup butter, room temperature
1 ⅔ cups white sugar
2 tablespoons cornstarch
1 tablespoon fresh lemon juice
1 tablespoon grated orange zest
2 teaspoons grated lime zest
1 ½ teaspoons grated lemon zest

1 ¼ cups all-purpose flour
½ teaspoon vanilla extract
3 eggs
1 cup sour cream
⅔ cup orange marmalade
2 teaspoons fresh lemon juice

Directions

1

Preheat oven to 450 degrees F. Butter a 9 inch springform pan. In a small bowl, whisk together egg yolk, 1 tablespoon lemon juice, 1 teaspoon lemon peel and 1/4 teaspoon vanilla. In the bowl of a food processor, combine flour and 1/3 cup sugar. Add butter and process until coarse crumbs form. With machine running, add yolk mixture and blend until moist clumps form. Press dough onto bottom and 1 1/2 inches up sides of prepared pan. Freeze crust 10 minutes.

2

Brush crust lightly with egg white. Bake until crust is pale golden, about 15 minutes. Cool on rack while preparing filling. Reduce oven temperature to 350 degrees F.

3

In a large bowl, beat cream cheese and 1 2/3 cups sugar until smooth. Beat in cornstarch, 1 tablespoon lemon juice, orange zest, lime zest, 1 1/2 teaspoon lemon zest and 1/2 teaspoon vanilla. Beat in eggs one at a time, then stir in sour cream. Pour filling into crust.

4

Bake in the preheated oven for 55 to 60 minutes, or until puffed and cracked around edges and center moves only slightly when pan is gently shaken. Allow to cool to room temperature, then refrigerate overnight.

5

In a saucepan over medium heat, boil marmalade and 2 teaspoons lemon juice until slightly reduced, about 2 minutes. Spread warm glaze on top of cake. Chill cake 10 minutes. Remove pan sides and transfer cake to serving plate.

Nutrition

Per Serving: 556 calories; protein 8.4g; carbohydrates 59.3g; fat 33g; cholesterol 153.9mg; sodium 263.6mg.

Strawberries Cream

Prep:

15 mins

Cook:

30 mins

Total:

45 mins

Servings:

12

Yield:

12 servings

Ingredients

½ cup butter, melted
1 cup milk
½ teaspoon salt
2 cups fresh strawberry halves
1 cup all-purpose flour
1 cup white sugar
2 teaspoons baking powder
1 (4 ounce) package cream cheese, cut into small pieces

Directions

1

Preheat oven to 400 degrees F.

2

Pour melted butter into the bottom of a 9x13-inch glass baking dish.

3

Mix milk, flour, sugar, baking powder, and salt together in a small bowl; pour over the butter in the baking dish. Arrange strawberry halves in a layer into the baking dish. Dot the strawberries with the cream cheese pieces.

4

Bake in preheated oven until top is golden brown and edges are bubbling, 30 to 40 minutes.

Nutrition

Per Serving: 222 calories; protein 2.7g; carbohydrates 28g; fat 11.5g; cholesterol 32.3mg; sodium 269.3mg.

Sweet Rice Pudding

Prep:

5 mins

Cook:

40 mins

Total:

45 mins

Servings:

4

Yield:

4 servings

Ingredients

1 ½ cups water

½ cup long grain rice

1 cup 2% milk

½ cup white sugar

1 tablespoon butter

1 pinch ground cinnamon

½ (12 fluid ounce) can evaporated milk

Directions

1

Bring water and rice to a boil in a saucepan. Reduce heat to medium-low, cover, and simmer until rice is tender and water has been absorbed, about 20. Add 2% milk, evaporated milk, sugar, and butter; stir well and cook until creamy, about 20 minutes longer. Serve sprinkled with cinnamon.

Nutrition

Per Serving: 301 calories; protein 6.9g; carbohydrates 51.3g; fat 7.8g; cholesterol 26.2mg; sodium 99.4mg.

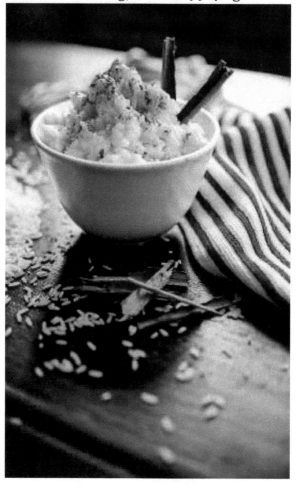

Brownie Pops

Prep:

30 mins

Cook:

38 mins

Additional:

1 hr 15 mins

Total:

2 hrs 23 mins

Servings:

36

Yield:

36 brownie pops

Ingredients

cooking spray

2 (18.3 ounce) packages fudge brownie mix (such as Duncan Hines®)

½ cup water

1 cup vegetable oil

4 eggs

Ganache:

6 ounces semisweet chocolate chips

1 (16 ounce) package confectioners' coating (such as Wilton® Candy Melts®)

½ cup heavy whipping cream

lollipop sticks

Directions

1

Preheat oven to 350 degrees F. Coat an 11x15-inch baking pan with cooking spray.

2

Empty brownie mix into a large bowl. Add vegetable oil, eggs, and water; stir with a wooden spoon until batter is well blended. Pour batter into the prepared baking pan.

3

Bake in the preheated oven until a toothpick inserted 1 inch from the edge of the pan comes out clean, 35 to 40 minutes. Let cool completely, about 30 minutes.

4

Combine chocolate chips and heavy cream in a microwave-safe bowl. Heat in the microwave in 30-second intervals, stirring after each interval, until melted and smooth. Cool, about 5 minutes.

5

Break brownies into pieces and place in a large bowl. Pour ganache evenly over brownie pieces; mix thoroughly.

6

Line a jelly roll pan with parchment paper. Press brownie mixture evenly into the pan. Freeze until firm, about 30 minutes.

7

Pour confectioners' coating into a microwave-safe bowl. Microwave at 50 percent power for 1 minute; stir thoroughly. Continue to microwave and stir at 30-second intervals until smooth and completely melted, 1 to 2 minutes more.

8

Roll brownie mixture into balls; insert a lollipop stick halfway into each. Dip balls one at a time into melted confectioners' coating to form a thin, even coating, letting the excess drip off. Stick into a styrofoam block; let stand until coating hardens, about 10 minutes.

Nutrition
Per Serving: 284 calories; protein 3.4g; carbohydrates 32.7g; fat 16.6g; cholesterol 28.6mg; sodium 132.6mg.

Black Forest

Servings:

18

Yield:

1 - 9 x 13 inch pan

Ingredients

1 (18.25 ounce) package devil's food cake mix with pudding
3 eggs
1 tablespoon butter
2 tablespoons milk
1 tablespoon almond extract
1 ½ cups semisweet chocolate chips
½ cup confectioners' sugar
1 (21 ounce) can cherry pie filling

Directions

1

Preheat oven to 350 degrees F.

2

Mix together: cake mix, beaten eggs, almond extract, cherry pie filling and 1 cup semisweet chocolate chips. Stir until just combined. Pour batter into a greased 9x13 inch pan.

3

Bake in a 350 degree F oven for 45 to 50 minutes or until a toothpick inserted in the center comes out clean. Remove cake from oven and let cool.

4

To Make Glaze: Heat 1/2 cup semisweet chocolate chips, butter or margarine, and milk in a saucepan over medium high heat. Once semisweet chocolate chips are melted and mixture is combined stir in confectioners' sugar.

5

Spread glaze over cooled cake. Serve cake as is or with whipped cream and a cherry.

Nutrition

Per Serving: 263 calories; protein 4.1g; carbohydrates 41.7g; fat 9.7g; cholesterol 38.5mg; sodium 235.7mg.

Pear Jam

Prep:

20 mins

Cook:

15 mins

Additional:

1 hr

Total:

1 hr 35 mins

Servings:

64

Yield:

8 half-pint jars

Ingredients

4 ½ cups mashed ripe pears
¼ cup lemon juice
7 ½ cups white sugar
1 teaspoon ground cinnamon
½ teaspoon ground cloves
½ teaspoon ground allspice
½ teaspoon ground nutmeg
1 teaspoon butter
8 half-pint canning jars with lids and rings
3 tablespoons powdered fruit pectin

Directions

1

Mix pears, fruit pectin, cinnamon, cloves, allspice, nutmeg, and lemon juice in a large heavy pot; bring to a boil, stirring constantly. Add sugar all at once, stirring, and bring back to a full rolling boil. Boil for 1 minute. Mix in butter to settle foam.

2

Sterilize the jars and lids in boiling water for at least 5 minutes. Pack the pear jam into the hot, sterilized jars, filling the jars to within 1/4 inch of the top. Run a knife or a thin spatula around the insides of the jars after they have been filled to remove any air bubbles. Wipe the rims of the jars with a moist paper towel to remove any food residue. Top with lids, and screw on rings.

3

Place a rack in the bottom of a large stockpot and fill halfway with water. Bring to a boil and lower jars into the boiling water using a holder. Leave a 2-inch space between the jars. Pour in more boiling water if necessary to bring the water level to at least 1 inch above the tops of the jars. Bring the water to a rolling boil, cover the pot, and process for 10 minutes.

4

Remove the jars from the stockpot and place onto a cloth-covered or wood surface, several inches apart, until cool. Once cool, press the top of each lid with a finger, ensuring that the seal is tight (lid does not move up or down at all). Store in a cool, dark area.

Nutrition

Per Serving: 99 calories; protein 0.1g; carbohydrates 25.4g; fat 0.1g; cholesterol 0.2mg; sodium 0.6mg.

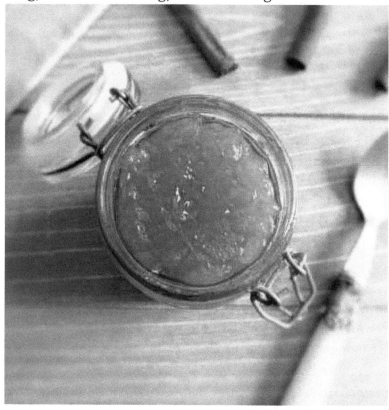

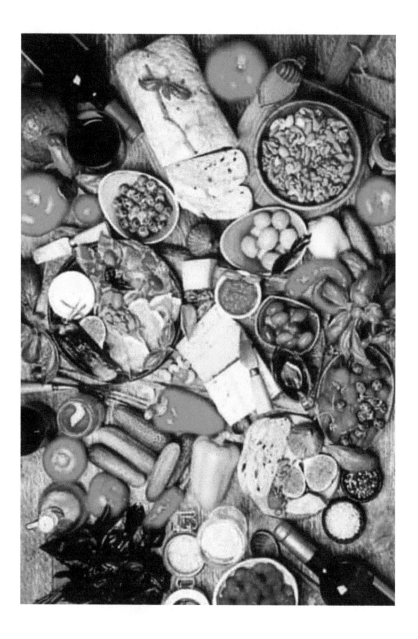

CPSIA information can be obtained
at www.ICGtesting.com
Printed in the USA
BVHW051946090421
604337BV00033B/670